The Beginner's Guide

TO A

HEALTHY LIFESTYLE

LARRY LEWIS

Disclaimer

The information contained in this guide is for educational purposes only and should not replace the care and/or advice of your doctor and healthcare providers.

Talk to your doctor before making any big changes to your diet or physical activity levels..

Contents

Welcome

In a nutshell a healthy lifestyle is all about making the right choices. You've made a wise choice by reading this book but that was the easy part. Whether you like it or not, you'll continue to make lifestyle choices from this moment forward, good and bad.

You have the choice to read through this guide right now and put the great information it contains to good use or you can simply ignore it and put it to one side to read later (and then forget about it never to be seen again).

My point? The conscious choices you make on a daily basis will determine if you live a healthy lifestyle or not!

A healthy lifestyle seems to be an incredibly popular topic. Due to its importance there should be no surprise with this. My blog gets a minimum of 500 people a day searching out information on a healthy lifestyle.

But, what I find crazy is how little people still know about a healthy lifestyle. Too many still seem not to know what it really means to have a healthy lifestyle or what they need to do.

When they start exploring to develop their understanding so they can make a start, they find themselves getting more and more confused by either conflicting information or in truth a lot of total nonsense people seem to write.

- Are you struggling with ill health?

- Maybe your doctor told you that you needed a healthier lifestyle.

- Maybe you're sick and tired of being the self-deprecating big guy/girl in your group of friends.

- Maybe you just had a child and realized you need to be there for him or her growing up.

- Maybe you woke up this morning, looked in the mirror, and finally came to the realization that it's time to start taking care of yourself.

Whatever your reason is for wanting to make a change, you're not alone! Every day, thousands of people make the decision to start improving their lifestyle...and every day those thousands of people don't really have any plan or idea what they're doing.

By the end of this guide you will no longer be in the dark.

But what does it really mean to have a healthy lifestyle?

First, let me make it very clear, a healthy lifestyle is far more than just diet and exercise.

In general, most would agree that a healthy person doesn't smoke, is at a healthy weight, eats a balanced healthy diet and exercises. Doing all four of these things would be a great start towards a healthy lifestyle, but there is more to it than that.

This guide is for people who are saying to themselves,

"I want to live a healthy life, but it seems so complicated; where should I begin?"

It is designed to help you successfully implement a healthier lifestyle. My goal is to put you in control of your health and to help you learn how to incorporate the necessary healthy lifestyle components into your and your family's lives.

To Your Health,

Larry Lewis.

Health & Wellness Life Coach.
www.healthylifestylesliving.com

About The Author

My Name Is Larry Lewis, Health & Wellness Life Coach, Blogger at Healthy Lifestyles Living, contributor to the Huffington Post, author of The Single Page Plan. Although originally from London I now live in County Durham, United Kingdom.

My life collapsed in 2009. I lost my amazing home, was declared bankrupt and life spiralled out of control having experienced extremely bad health, losing sight in one eye and the breakup of my marriage after 20 years. Probably nothing hurt me as much as the loss of my physique, muscles and fitness.

The journey back to fitness has been a hard one. Recovering from illness has been a rocky road. A journey I'm yet to fully complete, but now I am well on the road to making a full recovery, and have learnt so much more from being on the other side as they say. I am by far a better coach having now been on both sides of the fence, a gym instructor, healthy, and fit, and a guy struggling with ill health, unfit and fat.

I love to write, coach and inspire others. Being a qualified Life Coach, having owned my own chain of fitness clubs and having been a fitness instructor and someone who had been introduced to the field of personal development from the age of 13 and has studied and practiced it throughout my life, it was a natural progression to start a Wellness and Life Coaching practice and develop blogs, books and programs which allowed me to empower, and help others realise their personal health, fitness and life goals once I was no longer able to run my gyms after my loss of vision and retinal detachment.

I can help you. I don't have "magic answers" – there aren't any! I don't talk in jargon, psychobabble, or promote the latest big craze. I am straight forward and down to earth, with masses of experience backed up by qualifications, training and now life experiences. I use tried and tested techniques which I know work because they do for me!

We can all have health! With that being said, let's look at what it takes to have a healthy lifestyle.

It's so rewarding to see or hear stories about how many of my clients' and my readers lives have been transformed by the information I share. My purpose is to use my knowledge, experience, and enthusiasm to empower and inspire others to discover their passions and fulfil their dreams.

What Is A Healthy Lifestyle?

The starting point for this guide has to be to define exactly what is meant by the term a "healthy lifestyle.' To do this let's first look at the two words separately.

First we will define *HEALTH*.

THE WORLD HEALTH ORGANISATION IN 1946 DEFINED HEALTH AS:

"A complete state of mental, physical and social well-being not merely the absence of disease."

ACCORDING TO MERRIAM-WEBSTER THE DEFINITION OF HEALTH IS:

"The condition of being sound in body, mind, or spirit."

MY FAVOURITE DEFINITION IS FROM THE FREE DICTIONARY:

"A relative state in which one is able to function well physically, mentally, socially, and spiritually in order to express the full range of one's unique potentialities within the environment in which one is living."

Now let's look at the word *LIFESTYLE*. It is defined as "the way in which a person lives."

THE AMERICAN HERITAGE DICTIONARY OF THE ENGLISH LANGUAGE DEFINES LIFESTYLE AS:

"A way of life or style of living that reflects the attitudes and values of a person or group."

DICTIONARY.COM SAYS IT IS

"The habits, attitudes, tastes, moral standards, economic level, etc., that together constitute the mode of living of an individual or group."

WIKIPEDIA DEFINES A LIFESTYLE AS THE WAY A PERSON LIVES:

"This includes patterns of social relations, consumption, entertainment, and dress. A lifestyle typically also reflects an individual's attitudes, values or worldview. A healthy lifestyle is generally characterized as a balanced life in which one makes wise choices."

A FINAL DEFINITION OF LIFESTYLE IS:

"The aggregation of decisions by individuals which affect their health, and over which they more or less have control."

That's a whole lot of definitions but nowhere does any website (which I could find at the time of writing this guide) actually define the term "healthy lifestyle." So in the beginners guide spirit I have coined my own simple healthy lifestyle definition in one (easy to understand) sentence.

"A healthy lifestyle is making the best daily life choices to preserve good health and well-being, lowering the risk of being seriously ill or dying early."

Larry Lewis

Yes you did read that right. The risk of not having a healthy lifestyle is **death**. You may think I'm over exaggerating but it's so important to live a healthy lifestyle yet so many of us choose unhealthy lifestyle choices every day. We have the mindset of "it will never happen to me" but over time living an unhealthy lifestyle will catch up with all of us"

With that said, let's move on to the benefits of living a healthy lifestyle and how you can start making positive changes to your current lifestyle.

Benefits Of A Healthy Lifestyle

One thing that you all need to know, and that I am sure is a reason that many of you are here is that although not all illnesses are preventable, it is a fact that a large proportion of deaths, particularly those from coronary heart disease and lung cancer, can be avoided. In addition many chronic diseases can also be avoided. Both of these things can be achieved by having a healthy lifestyle. Can there be anything more important?

To those of you going through illness right now, you have my sympathies. I know how hard a time like this can be. I do hope you are getting great support from others. I know I have a lot of doctors to thank for part of my recovery but, and this is a big but, much of my recovery wasn't me relying exclusively on the care I was getting from the highly trained health professionals and doctors but it was down to me making big changes in my lifestyle.

You owe it to yourself to create a lifestyle that is going to best support you and ultimately help you recuperate. A healthy lifestyle can help bring about dramatic improvements as well as ensuring things don't get worse.

To those of you who have no health worries in the slightest, do everything you can to ensure things stay as they are and your best way of preventing problems in the future is by having a healthy lifestyle today.

Every one of you has your own motivations for wanting to start building your own healthy lifestyle. I'm sure we all want to live a long, happy and healthy life where we are always full of energy and vitality, free from disease and illness.

There are plenty more reasons why having a healthy lifestyle is a good idea.

- A healthy lifestyle has an incredible number of benefits, for example:

- Reduces the incidence and impact of health problems

- Reduce the risk of heart disease, stroke and diabetes

- Reduction in probability of virtually all diseases

- Increase the length of one's life

- Improve joint stability and flexibility

- Increase overall strength and stamina

- Maintain bone density

- Prevent osteoporosis and bone fractures

- Improve sense of wellness and mood

- Reduce symptoms of anxiety and depression

- Improve self-esteem

- Improved self-confidence

- Improve sharpness and clarity of mind

- Improve memory in elderly people

- Reduce stress

- *Improves our quality of life*

Let me back this up with a few statistics, just to ensure you truly understand the importance of having a healthy lifestyle.

The NHS (National Health Service - UK) annually spends more than:

- £5 billion on obesity-related conditions

- £2.7 billion on alcohol-related conditions

Both of which are the result of lifestyle choices impacting on an individual's health.

In a report discussing these statistics it was said:

"As a measure to improve the health of the nation, and the resources and sustainability of the NHS, it would be advantageous to explore ways in which an individual's lifestyle choices could be changed to promote health and prevent lifestyle related diseases burdening the NHS."

Source: 2013 Scottish Universities Medical Journal

The Health Survey for England 2011 found:

- Obesity has increased substantially over the period of 1993 to 2011 from 13% to 24% in men and 16% to 26% in women.

- 23% of adults are obese with a BMI of over 30 and 61% are overweight or obese with a BMI greater than 25.

- 33% of 10- 11 year olds and 23% of 4-5 year olds also have a BMI greater than 25.

- In 2010, obesity was responsible for 11,173 episodes of treatment in hospitals equating to 25,322 bed days with a mean stay in hospital of 3.7 days.

- If current trends in obesity remain, the estimated annual cost to the NHS in 2015 for diseases related to being overweight and obesity amount to £15 billion with obesity alone predicted to demand £9 billion.

- Doctor-diagnosed diabetes increased in men from 2.9% in 1993 to 7% in 2011, and 1.9% to 4.9% in women over the same time period.

- It is estimated there are 2.8 million people with diabetes and it is predicted to increase to 4 million by 2025.

- The rise in obesity is predicted to correlate with a rise in diabetes prevalence of 6-8.5 million and 5.7-7.3 million cases of stroke and heart disease.

It drew the conclusion that:

"More needs to be done to change the attitudes and behaviours of individuals to lifestyle choices in order to promote health and prevent disease, consequently easing the strain on NHS services and resources that is currently imposed upon them."

Compelling evidence for the importance of a healthy lifestyle!

Now let me share some good news. An overweight person by achieving a proper weight level can:

- Cut their risk of heart disease by up to 25%,

- Reduce their risk of a heart attack by 29%,

- Reduce their risk of diabetes by up to 64%,

- Reduce their risk of having high cholesterol by 33%,

- Reduce their risk of dying from any cause by 16%,

- Reduce their risk of asthma by 30%,

- Reduce their risk of stomach cancer by 10%,

- Reduce their risk of gallstones by 60%,

- Cut their risk of osteoarthritis by 12%,

- Reduce their risk of oesophageal cancer by 55%,

- Cut their risk of having high blood pressure by 44%.

So what do all these stats and figures really mean? In a nutshell we are living life today without a thought for the future. Too many unhealthy conveniences are taking precedence over good healthy choices. After all it takes less time to phone for a takeaway than stand and cook a healthy meal right? Unfortunately our mindset is one that will happily choose convenience and more time over health and wellbeing.

If you don't want to become a statistic then surely you only have one choice - **to now start implementing a healthy lifestyle.**

It Comes Down To Choice

Every day we get to make choices.

Some of these choices are insignificant, like which socks you are going to put on in the morning.

Others can change your life forever, for example deciding that you will never smoke again.

Whatever choices we make we have to accept the consequences of them whether good or bad.

If you have from this point forward chosen to live a healthy lifestyle, it is your responsibility to follow through on this. What I will ensure is you know the things that you're going to have to do.

Let's be clear here. Living a healthy, happy life depends on you implementing a healthy lifestyle. Implementing a healthy lifestyle depends on the choices you make.

Let's look at a few obvious examples.

- You choose to spend your free time today watching Television *or alternatively you choose to spend one hour in the gym.*

- You choose to eat a greasy fry up for breakfast *or alternatively you choose oatmeal and fruit.*

- Every time you're thirsty you choose to drink coca cola *or alternatively you choose water.*

- After a difficult meeting you choose to drown your sorrows with alcohol *or alternatively you spend 30 minutes unwinding and relaxing through meditation.*

You see everything in life *gives you alternatives*, and you're completely free to make your choice about which alternative you take. But remember every action has a reaction, or in other words, when you choose an action, you choose the consequences of that action.

Only you can make good lifestyle choices in order to achieve what is surely your number one life goal – to enjoy good health.

So are you ready to make the right choices and to implement a healthy lifestyle?

If you are this guide is going to show you exactly the type of lifestyle you need to build. It will require some work, but your health is well worth the investment!

So let us move on to show you the dos and don'ts of a healthy lifestyle.

How Healthy Are You Now

How good have your choices been so far? Are you making good healthy lifestyle choices on a regular basis or are you on a path to obesity and illness?

Go and take my healthy lifestyle quiz (https://www.healthylifestylesliving.com/health/healthy-lifestyle/healthy-lifestyle-quiz/) now, this guide will still be here when you get back. The central aspect of this assessment is our 15-points lifestyle formula, which quickly and accurately highlights areas of strength and weaknesses. It enables you to assess where you are on a healthy lifestyle scale. In a simple and non-intrusive way, you will quickly determine how healthy your lifestyle is.

Don't get too caught up on your score for now. If it's low then there is room for improvement and if it's high, don't get too smug because it only takes a few bad habits to sneak into your daily routine to destroy that nice high score.

The point of this quiz is to provide you with a starting point.

The Components of a Healthy Lifestyle

Ok, it's time to buckle up and hold on to your hat! I'm going to show you the do's and don'ts for achieving a healthy lifestyle.

This section is looong and it contains an amazing amount of tips, techniques and general information but don't panic! I don't expect you to change things over night and become a healthy lifestyle master just by reading this beginners guide.

It's been crafted to get you started on a healthy lifestyle. Like the title says, it will provide a great starting point for someone who is looking to explore what a healthy lifestyle really entails. Don't worry though I won't leave you hanging! At the end of this guide, I will show you how you can get more advanced training on the topics I'm about to cover now.

Here's what not to do.

DON'T MAKE EXCUSES

Do you have excuses for not having a healthy lifestyle? At the beginning of every year many of you always set out to bring about big changes in your life. Often these changes will include things like losing weight, getting into shape, improving fitness. Alas often before even the end of January you fall off the wagon and find all the excuses you can for why you just can't do it.

It's so common to make excuses to just why you can't build a healthy lifestyle and as a former gym owner I've heard them all.

- It's just so difficult – *yes it can be hard to put years of bad habits behind you, but the results will be worth every struggle.*

- I'm ok at the moment - *Maybe you are, but don't wait till things force you to change.*

- I've never had a day sick in my life - *Now then is the perfect time to focus on embracing healthy habits that will keep you feeling that way; do not wait until you're sick to live a healthy lifestyle*

- My work schedule makes living a healthy lifestyle impossible - *You can't put your work or your to-do-list before your personal health all the time.*

- I'm not ready to make a change – *there's never a right time to start, but surely its best to make the changes needed before ill health sets in.*

- I find temptations are too great - *Staying in bed instead of going to the gym can be tempting, as maybe that bar of chocolate is asking you to eat it. Then sleep in or eat that bar of chocolate. You've surely heard of the 80 -20 theory. Live that healthy lifestyle 80% of the time and you'll be doing ok as far as I'm concerned.*

- What if it doesn't work out? *Creating a healthy lifestyle is possible if you are committed and stay focused, and your health is too important to fail with this.*

- I can eat, drink and live a lazy sedentary life and don't put on weight or seem to suffer with bad health - *Not yet anyway. Doomsday may be just round the corner, so stop it before it does.*

- A healthy lifestyle costs too much – *I believe you'll find takeaways aren't cheap, nor is alcohol; chocolate and cakes aren't free and ill health can be incredibly expensive in many ways.*

- I'm too old - *It's never too late to take care of your health. And before you start, no matter how overweight, out of shape, inflexible, too flexible, old, young, or ailing body you may have, a healthy lifestyle will help you get fitter, healthier and happy with who you are.*

I'm sure you can think of other excuses that you've used for not having a healthy lifestyle, but now this is the time where you're going to do it. No excuses will ever stand in the way of someone totally committed. After all ultimately we are talking about the difference between possibly life and death.

DON'T SMOKE

It causes things such as respiratory illness, coronary heart disease, cancer.

Your family's risks are increased two to three times if you smoke.

If you are pregnant you can damage your baby's chances of being healthy by smoking even before the baby is born.

Research shows that young children who have one or more parents who smoke are twice as likely to suffer with chest problems in their first year of life. They will have more chest, nose, ear and throat infections than children whose parents do not smoke. They are also more likely to take up smoking themselves later in life.

Smoking kills around 120,000 people prematurely in the UK every year - more than 13 people every hour. It is also responsible for many diseases, including cancers, heart disease and stroke.

I could go on and on about the dangers of smoking.

The only thing I cannot give you is a single benefit or good reason for smoking.

This is very simple, smoking is incredibly bad for you.

You want a healthy lifestyle you can't smoke, SIMPLE!

If you don't smoke, then don't start. If you do smoke you can lower your health risks by stopping. Talk to your doctor about medicines to help you quit or to find out about Nicotine Replacement Therapy.

The health benefits will start immediately once you quit smoking.

Let's be clear here – **To have a healthy lifestyle you can't smoke!**

DON'T DRINK TO EXCESS

Here is the good news for some of you. I'm not advocating never drinking alcohol. I will hold my hands up to enjoying the occasional glass of red wine.

Indeed there is a lot of research which suggests drinking small quantities of alcohol can reduce the risk of heart disease.

However as the amount and number of times a week you drink increases, then so do the risks.

My suggestion is if you aren't a drinker don't start. If you are then limit your amounts to lower the health risks.

To keep health risks from alcohol to a low level, the UK Chief Medical Officers' (CMO) advised that it is safest not to drink more than 14 units a week on a regular basis.

One unit is 10ml of pure alcohol. Because alcoholic drinks come in different strengths and sizes units are a good way of telling how strong your drink is. It's not as simple as one drink, one unit.

The new alcohol unit guidelines are equivalent to six pints of average strength beer or six 175ml glasses of average strength wine.

As I will emphasis shortly, water is a far better choice of drink.

DON'T DRINK COFFEE TO EXCESS

Ok I'll be honest, this was one of my hardest challenges. I'm a coffee addict. I simply love sitting in Costa or Starbucks coffee shops writing my articles. Simply Heaven. But as they say too much of a good thing isn't actually good for you.

Studies do show that drinking coffee can lower risk of diseases like type 2 diabetes, neurological disorders and liver diseases. So in the right amounts it's definitely good for you.

However, just because a little bit of something is good, it doesn't mean that too much will be as well.

Again I'm not saying you have to cut out coffee or tea entirely. But you do have to limit your consumption.

In its guidelines on caffeine consumption, the EU's food safety watchdog has advised a daily limit of 400mg. This equates to about 4 cups of coffee.

What I will say is Green Tea is an excellent option if you are looking for a hot and healthy beverage.

There of course are other Don't Do's if you want a healthy lifestyle. Unprotected sex with a stranger would be one thing not to do. Driving without a seat belt. Taking recreational drugs. I would say these are things that just a little bit of common sense would say don't do them.

So with the lecture over let's now take a look at what you need to do in order to achieve and live a healthy lifestyle. Remember this list has been simplified to keep this guide compact and easy to consume. Again, for those who would like to go in to more advanced detail on these topics then at the end of this guide I will provide you with some links on how to get more advanced information.

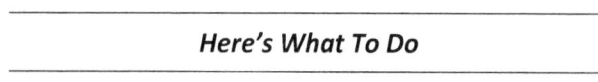

Here's What To Do

TAKE ONE STEP AT A TIME

Rome wasn't built in a day. If you try and make every change immediately that's necessary for you to have a healthy lifestyle you're setting yourself up for failure. I want you to succeed. I want you to have a healthy lifestyle and enjoy the good health that will come from that. So what we have found is those implementing one or two changes at a time are those who will be successful. They allow these changes to bed in before making another change or two.

I'm going to make quite a few suggestions from this point forward, many of which will be the complete opposite to what you're doing currently. There is no doubt that you will have some bad habits. These have been with you for probably as long as you can remember. They are pretty much ingrained into your psyche. So to change them is going to be hard for you. By being able to concentrate on creating just one or two new habits at a time is going to help you keep focused on them which will result in you eliminating for ever your bad habits and replacing them with really good ones.

BE AT A HEALTHY WEIGHT

Your current lifestyle, whether it is good or bad, can, to a point, be demonstrated by your current weight. A healthy weight indicates that you have a good lifestyle where being overweight would indicate you have a bad lifestyle as would being under weight.

Whether it is a good indication or not, if you weigh too much or too little it certainly can be bad for your health. It can even cause serious conditions, such as heart disease and cancer. Therefore, it's a good idea to keep an eye on your weight to make sure you stay within a healthy range.

Statistics show in England alone, nearly a quarter of men and women are now obese. Being obese specifically refers to having an excess amount of body fat. The trends for children give even more cause for concern, with 18 per cent of 2 to 15 year olds currently obese and a further 14 per cent overweight. The Foresight report on obesity indicated that nearly 60 per cent of the UK population could be obese by 2050.

As dangerous as it is to carry around extra weight, being underweight is also associated with a higher mortality rate. Being underweight can lead to the malfunctioning of many important body functions. It can also result in a loss of energy and an increased susceptibility to injury, infection, and illness.

Genetics, environment, social, behavioural, and psychological reasons can all be factors in an abnormal body weight. You may not be able to change some of these factors, but one you can change is your lifestyle habits. Taking a few simple steps can make all the difference. If you're overweight, losing even a few pounds will make a positive difference to your health.

The first things you should measure are your BMI, your waist circumference and your waist-to-hip ratio. Check out my free weights and measurements tool which you can use to calculate these measurements for you.

HAVE AN ACTIVE LIFESTYLE

People who don't get enough physical activity are much more likely to develop health problems.

Regular, moderate-intensity aerobic physical activity can lower your risk of:

- Heart disease and heart attack

- High blood pressure

- High total cholesterol, high LDL (bad) cholesterol and low HDL (good) cholesterol

- Overweight or obesity

- Diabetes

- Stroke

There are many ways each one of you can have a more active lifestyle. Whether you are a busy mum or dad, young or old, an office or factory worker, or whatever it is you do, you can build physical activity into your life. In this particular case I'm not referring to fitness, or sports, but in its far simplest term, getting busy using and moving your body.

Everybody, regardless of age, shape, size and ability needs to become more active every day. We should all be moving more incorporating activity into our daily life.

We know that, at both work and home, technology encourages us to sit for long periods. We are also more likely to use motorised transport rather than walking or cycling, or use lifts instead of stairs. Well buck the trend. Find ways to get yourself active.

Try not to sit for hours on end. I suggest in every hour you get up and walk around for between 5 – 10 minutes.

You can benefit from moderate activities like these:

- Brisk walking

- Walk to the local shops instead of drive, or take the dog for a walk.

- Hand washing/waxing a car

- Actively playing with children

- Gardening and yard work

- Moderate to heavy housework

- Take the stairs instead of lifts and escalators.

- Pleasure dancing and home exercise

More vigorous physical activity can further improve the fitness of your heart and lungs which we will look at in the next component of a healthy lifestyle.

Making small changes in your lifestyle can make a big difference in your overall health. Stop thinking about living an active lifestyle in terms of workouts and exercise, and start thinking about in terms of **living life!**

INCLUDE FITNESS AS PART OF YOUR LIFE

You will need to include fitness as part of your life. Physical fitness keeps your weight in check, helps you sleep better at night, prevents heart attacks and strokes and other health problems, and generally prolongs your life. Basically there are so many benefits of exercising that you really can't live a full life without it.

Physical fitness is necessary to stimulate the body's own natural maintenance and repair system. Your bones, joints and muscles – especially your heart – will actually stay younger if you keep them busy. If you are not Physically Active you increase your Health Risks in many ways.

There are so many risks to not having a reasonable level of physical fitness.

Coronary heart disease, strokes, high blood pressure, breathlessness, flabby body, little energy, stiff joints, osteoporosis, poor posture, overweight.

You need to find opportunities to develop *STAMINA, STRENGTH* and *SUPPLENESS*.

STAMINA: You need a well-developed circulation to the heart and lungs to give you the ability to keep going without gasping for breath. With stamina you have a slower, more powerful heartbeat and will be able to cope more easily with prolonged or heavy exercise. You need to introduce *CARIOVASCULAR EXERCISE*. Choose aerobics, running, swimming, brisk walking, dancing ... you have so many choices.

STRENGTH: You need well-toned muscles to give you the ability to do physical work. When your shoulder, trunk and thigh muscles are toned-up they will work well and you will not experience strains and injuries as often. *YOU NEED TO INTRODUCE WEIGHT TRAINING* of some description.

SUPPLENESS: Developing good mobility in your neck, spine and joints will prevent you spraining ligaments and pulling muscles and tendons. You will also be less likely to experience aches and pains from stiff joints. *YOU NEED TO INTRODUCE STRETCHING.*

If you are already physically active continue being so and use more variety of movement. If not, start slowly and don't do too much too soon. Listen to your body: if you experience dizziness, nausea, pain and extreme tiredness you are doing too much too soon.

If you are comfortable with what you are doing increase the amount of exercise and *BUILD IT UP GRADUALLY.*

According to guidelines from the UK Chief Medical Officer, we should aim to take part in at least 150 minutes of moderate intensity physical activity each week, in bouts of 10 minutes or more.

So aim for half an hour of *MODERATELY INTENSE* Physical Activity *FIVE* or more days a week.

MODERATELY INTENSE Physical Activity means you should get slightly out of breath. This is healthy. If your muscles are working better so is your heart.

What you will achieve:

You will be *LESS* at risk from major illnesses and minor ailments such as colds. You will have *MORE ENERGY* to spend on living. You will *FEEL HEALTHIER*.

HEALTHY EATING

Healthy eating is an essential part of leading a healthy lifestyle. Your body requires a well-balanced diet every day in order to maintain the adequate amounts of vitamins, nutrients and minerals needed to maintain a healthy weight and body as well as protect you from certain diseases.

"To eat is a necessity, but to eat intelligently is an art"

- La Rochefoucauld (French Writer)

A nutrient is anything in food that:

- Provides energy

- Helps your body "burn" another nutrient to provide energy

- Helps build or repair tissue

Making healthy choices can sometimes be hard, but there are easy changes you can make to eat better. To help prevent heart disease, stroke, and perhaps other diseases, you should eat mainly:

Fruit: Adults should eat between 1½ to 2 cups of fruit every day. Fruit is great for a snack, side item or dessert (like one small banana, one large orange, and ¼ cup of dried apricots or peaches).

Vegetables: Adults should eat 2½ to 3 cups of vegetables per day. Try to pick a variety of colours when selecting veggies at the store. Eat more dark green veggies (such as broccoli, kale, spinach, and other dark leafy greens); orange veggies (like sweet potatoes or carrots); and beans and peas.

Protein: Adults should eat 5 to 6 ounces of protein per day. Choose lean meat, poultry, and fish. Mix up your protein sources with more beans, peas, nuts, and seeds, as well as eggs. Fish is a great option. Broil, bake, steam, or grill it. Fish and shellfish contain a type of fat called omega-3 fatty acids — it's good for you! Research suggests that eating omega-3 fatty acids lowers your chances of dying from heart disease. Fish that naturally contain more oil (such as salmon, trout, herring, mackerel, anchovies, and sardines) have more omega-3 fatty acids than lean fish (such as cod, haddock, and catfish).

Grains: Adults should eat 5 to 7 ounces of grains per day. Choose whole grains like whole wheat bread and pasta, brown rice, oatmeal and whole wheat cereal instead of refined (white) grains whenever possible. One ounce is about one slice of bread, 1 cup of breakfast cereal, or ½ cup of cooked rice or pasta. Eat at least 3 ounces of whole-grain cereals, breads, crackers, rice, or pasta every day. Eat whole-wheat bread instead of white bread or brown rice instead of white rice.

Dairy: Adults should eat less than 3 servings of low-fat dairy (milk, yogurt, cheese) per day. Fat-free or low-fat versions of milk, cheese, yogurt, and other milk products.

You can avoid unhealthy foods by limiting:

Saturated fat (Saturated fat is the main dietary cause of high blood cholesterol. It is found mostly in foods from animals and some plants.)

Trans fat (The amount of trans fat content in foods is printed on the Nutrition Facts label. Keep trans fat intake to less than 1 percent of total calories. For example, if you need 2,000 calories a day, you should consume less than 2 grams of trans fat.)

Cholesterol

Sodium. Limit salt. Eat less than 2,300 mg of sodium (about 1 teaspoon of salt) each day. If you are older than age 51, or if you are African-American (at any age), or if you have hypertension, diabetes, or chronic kidney disease, you should eat less than 1,500 mg of sodium each day. Most of the salt we eat each day actually comes from processed foods rather than salt that we add to foods that we cook. Cut back on frozen dinners, pizza, packaged mixes, canned soups or broths, and salad dressings — these often have a lot of sodium. Make sure to check the sodium content on the Nutrition Facts label when buying food.

Added sugars. Since sugars contribute calories with few, if any, nutrients, look for foods and beverages low in added sugars. Read the ingredient list and make sure that added sugars are not one of the first few ingredients. Some names for added sugars include sucrose, glucose, high fructose corn syrup, corn syrup, maple syrup, and fructose.

To stay at a healthy weight, you need to balance the calories you eat with the calories you use up (burn). To lose weight, you need to burn more calories than you eat. A healthy diet and physical activity can help you control your weight.

GET ENOUGH SLEEP

Shakespeare described sleep as "the chief nourisher in life's feast", acknowledging that for most of us deep rest is necessary for keeping body, mind and spirit in good form.

Getting enough sleep is vital if you want to live a healthy lifestyle.

A lack of sleep has been linked to various problems, including:

- Greater risk of depression and anxiety

- Increased risk of heart disease and cancer

- Impaired memory

- Reduced immune system functioning

- Weight gain

- Greater likelihood of accidents

Getting enough continuous quality sleep contributes to how we feel and perform the next day, but also has a huge impact on the overall quality of our lives. Getting enough sleep refers to the amount of sleep you need to feel rested and alert the next day. Most sleep experts recommend 7-9 hours of sleep per night. Although some people can get along with less sleep, others find they need as much as 10 hours per night to feel rested the next day.

To try and ensure your best night sleep possible:

- Give yourself at least 30 minutes relaxation period before bedtime so to disengage your mind.

- Ensure your bedroom is not too warm and has good air circulation

- Empty your bladder before going to bed

- Do not drink a very large amount of any beverage too close to bedtime, which will cause you to wake to empty your bladder, thus disturbing your rest.

- Preparation for the next day long before bedtime can help to reduce apprehension

- Keep a window slightly open to allow fresh air to enter your bedroom

MAINTAIN PERSONAL HYGIENE

Maintaining good personal hygiene is another important step for a healthy lifestyle. Personal hygiene involves those practices performed by an individual to care for one's bodily health and well-being, through cleanliness.

Good personal hygiene can help you ward off illnesses and certainly prevents them from getting any worse. I have seen too many people when ill stopping taking care of themselves, not washing, bathing or changing clothes. In consequence to this their conditions have worsened and other problems developed.

Practising good body hygiene also helps us to feel good about our self, which is also important for our mental health.

Proper personal hygiene is essential for social interactions and respect in the professional arena as people who have poor hygiene (body odour, bad breath, etc) often are seen as unhealthy and may face discrimination.

The steps below will help you to improve personal hygiene:

- Bathe or Shower regularly. Wash your body and your hair often.

- Trim your nails.

- Brush and floss your teeth.

- Wash your hands.

- Take care of your hair.

- Wear Clean Clothes.

- Keep your living environment clean and tidy.

- Keep bacteria, viruses, and illnesses at bay.

DRINK PLENTY OF WATER

Water is essential to a healthy lifestyle.

Cut out or reduce the sodas, beers, sports drinks and cordials. Instead drink water, lots of it.

Most of you probably don't *drink enough* water.

Without water, you will die. When you don't take enough of it, your performance and results will suffer.

Water is essential for our body to function. It is involved in all metabolic processes. It helps everything from electrolyte balance to hydration, digestion, metabolism, kidney health, lower incidence of urinary infection and protein synthesis.

When we are properly hydrated our heart and blood vessels work much better, along with all of our other bodily functions—we think better, our strength and endurance are better, we feel better, we are healthier, and we will live longer.

- Do you know over 60% of our body is made up of water?

Water is needed by every living cell and almost every process that takes place within the body is dependent on water.

The body uses about 10 - 12 cups of water a day, through such things as breathing, digestion, elimination and perspiration. So we need to replenish it daily or our bodies will become dehydrated. It is required for digestion and absorption of food. It is needed to regulate body temperature and blood circulation. Water in the bloodstream carries nutrients and oxygen to cells. It is necessary for the kidneys to remove toxins and other wastes. Since we lose water every day through urine, bowel movements, perspiration and breathing, we need to replenish our water intake.

Aim to drink at least 2 litres every single day.

I carry around with me a water bottle and refill it 3 or 4 times throughout the day.

PRACTICE STRESS MANAGEMENT

Emotional stress is responsible for a huge range of physical and mental illness so stress management is an essential part of a healthy lifestyle.

"Diseases of the soul are more dangerous and more numerous than those of the body."

- Marcus Tullius Cicero (Roman Philosopher)

Stress Management can be defined as interventions designed to reduce the impact of stressors in your life giving you the individual more of an ability to cope with the stressors you face. The goal of Stress Management is to help you to manage the stress of everyday life.

Stress management as described in Wikipedia, the free encyclopedia refers to a wide spectrum of techniques and psychotherapies aimed at controlling a person's levels of stress, especially chronic stress, usually for the purpose of improving everyday functioning.

It's a simple, unavoidable fact that stress is a part of most people's lives.

It is a reality that we all live with.

Yet stress management exists to help us reduce its impact upon us greatly.

Managing stress to me is a huge part of promoting healthy lifestyle living. There are so many simple and effective ways to handle stress and improve health, both mentally and physically so it makes total sense to take action and do something to get your stress in check.

Reducing stress in your everyday life is vital for maintaining your overall health, as it can improve your mood, boost immune function, promote longevity and allow you to be more productive. When you let your stress get the best of you, you put yourself at risk of developing a range of illnesses – from the common cold to severe heart disease. Stress has such a powerful impact on your well-being because it is a natural response that is activated in the brain. Let's examine how this process works, why stress affects you the way it does, and the severe impacts it can have on your health.

When faced with a threat, the body's defence's kick into the "fight-or-flight" response. The body calls upon all its forces to confront the oncoming threat and protect you from harm. It's your body's defence mechanism, resulting in the following reactions:

- Heartbeat increases; pumping blood to the necessary parts of the body quickly.

- Blood pressure increases

Blood flow:

- Is constricted to the digestive organs.

- Increases to the brain and major organs.

- Increases to the major muscles.

- Constricted to the extremities e.g. hands and feet

- Muscles tense up

- Breathing becomes more shallow and rapid.

- Your nervous system releases stress hormones such as Adrenaline into the bloodstream.

- Blood loss in case of injury is prevented by your Blood vessels constricting

- Your Pupils dilate allowing more light in and other senses become heightened

- The liver releases stored sugar into the blood stream

- Other non-essential body processes are suppressed.

- Your digestive system is slowed down, as is your reproductive system

- Growth hormones are turned off.

- Your immune response is repressed.

- The body perspires

- Metabolic rate increases

- Blood clotting agents are released.

Thankfully it does stop short of turning you into The Incredible Hulk!

These stress responses are there to protect and support us and have their uses, in the right circumstances, particularly life-or-death situations. They help us to fight with more strength or run away faster.

In the world we find ourselves in today, most of our stress is brought on by psychological threats, not physical ones; it's just that our minds and bodies can't tell the difference. The stress response will be activated over an approaching deadline, an argument with the wife, a mass of unpaid bills, your teenage daughter being late home, your petrol warning light flashing on a country road. So no differently to a caveman confronting a dinosaur, our bodies go into this automatic response.

The more frequently our stress response is activated, the harder it is to turn it off. Instead of subsiding once an emergency has gone, our stress hormones, and increased heart rate and blood pressure remain high. This in turn takes a heavy toll on the body.

The risk to your health, and threat of serious illness, is increased dramatically through this constant exposure to stress. That is why learning to deal with stress is essential for you, learning tools and techniques that will help you handle stress in a positive way, and thereby reducing the harmful impact that stress has on your life.

When stress is in control of you, it also controls your attitude to life and your physical health.

"Stress is not what happens to us. It's our response to what happens. And response is something we can choose."

- Maureen Killoran

Stress comes from our internal perception of the world and the things that we perceive to be threatening to us.

Having a certain amount of pressure in our lives is good. It gets us going. What is important is keeping the pressures on you at the right level. Too much pressure, on a constant basis doesn't allow you recovery time, and can result in health problems. So is it surprising that so many people now suffer from stress? There is no stigma to being diagnosed as suffering from stress, it's now so common. There is no divide, no class distinction; it's the price many of us are paying for modern living.

Stress, we know, when it gets too much will cause physical and emotional problems, as well as ill health. Through my healthy lifestyle blog I give you the tools and techniques to manage stress effectively.

Managing stress is such an overlooked part of being able to live a healthy lifestyle. We concentrate more on how we look that how we feel but manage stress we must. I've already gone on way to long about stress in this guide but there is so much more to cover so for now I will leave you with these articles from my healthy lifestyle blog which you can read in your own time. They contain great advice and stress management techniques which you can use to keep your stress levels in check.

STRESS MANAGEMENT ARTICLES

8 Relaxation Techniques That You Can Use Daily (https://www.healthylifestylesliving.com/enlighten-the-soul/stress-management/8-relaxation-techniques-that-you-can-use-daily/)

Relaxation Technique One Deep Breathing
(https://www.healthylifestylesliving.com/enlighten-the-soul/relaxation-technique-one-deep-breathing/)
Relaxation Technique Two Progressive Muscular Relaxation
(https://www.healthylifestylesliving.com/enlighten-the-soul/stress-management/relaxation-technique-2-progressive-muscular-relaxation/)
Relaxation Technique Three Meditation
(https://www.healthylifestylesliving.com/enlighten-the-soul/relaxation-technique-three-meditation/)
Relaxation Technique Four Visualisation
(https://www.healthylifestylesliving.com/enlighten-the-soul/stress-management/relaxation-technique-four-visualisation/)
Relaxation Technique Five Get Into Centre
(https://www.healthylifestylesliving.com/enlighten-the-soul/stress-management/relaxation-technique-five-get-into-centre/)
Relaxation Technique Six Mental Imagery
(https://www.healthylifestylesliving.com/enlighten-the-soul/stress-management/relaxation-technique-six-mental-imagery/)
Stop Stressing... I said Stop
(https://www.healthylifestylesliving.com/enlighten-the-soul/stress-management/stop-stressing-i-said-stop/)
The Long Road of Parenting 10 Tips for Your Journey
(https://www.healthylifestylesliving.com/enlighten-the-soul/stress-management/the-long-road-of-parenting-10-stress-tips-for-your-journey/)
Start to Reduce your Stress
(https://www.healthylifestylesliving.com/enlighten-the-soul/stress-management/start-to-reduce-your-stress/)

In today's world, it's becoming ever harder to escape the effects of stress. So, use these articles to learn the techniques that can help you cope with stress. Enjoy the relaxing benefits.

POWERING UP YOUR MIND

Healthy people differ significantly in their overall personality, mood, and behaviour. Each person also varies from day to day, depending on the circumstances. However, a sudden, major change in personality and/or behaviour, particularly one that is not related to an obvious event (such as taking a drug or losing a loved one), often indicates a problem.

Your mental health influences how you think, feel, and behave in daily life. It also affects your ability to cope with stress, overcome challenges, build relationships, and recover from life's setbacks and hardships. Whether you're looking to cope with a specific mental health problem, handle your emotions better, or simply to feel more positive and energetic, there are plenty of things you can do to take control of your mental health—starting today.

Programme your mind for total success. Develop a vision, a compelling future that excites and inspires you, and focus on it daily. Don't let anything knock you of course, or make you question its possibility. I promise you, by taking control of your thoughts, you will improve your life in a big way.

"In minds crammed with thoughts, organs clogged with toxins, and bodies stiffened with neglect, there is just no space for anything else"

- Alison Rose Levy (Journalist)

Mental health refers to your overall psychological well-being. It includes the way you feel about yourself, the quality of your relationships, and your ability to manage your feelings and deal with difficulties.

Good mental health isn't just the absence of mental health problems. Being mentally or emotionally healthy is much more than being free of depression, anxiety, or other psychological issues. Rather than the absence of mental illness, mental health refers to the presence of positive characteristics.

People who are mentally healthy have:

- A sense of contentment

- A zest for living and the ability to laugh and have fun.

- The ability to deal with stress and bounce back from adversity.

- A sense of meaning and purpose, in both their activities and their relationships.

- The flexibility to learn new things and adapt to change.

- A balance between work and play, rest and activity, etc.

- The ability to build and maintain fulfilling relationships.

- Self-confidence and high self-esteem.

These positive characteristics of mental and emotional health allow you to participate in life to the fullest extent possible through productive, meaningful activities and strong relationships. These positive characteristics also help you cope when faced with life's challenges and stresses.

BE AT PEACE WITH THE WORLD - SPIRITUALLY

What is spiritual health? The word "spiritual" refers to that core dimension of you - your innermost self - that provides you with a profound sense of who you are, where you came from, where you're going and how you might reach your goal.

Spiritual health is a highly individualized concept that is measured by the amount of peace and harmony an individual experiences in his day-to-day life.

You may not think much about spiritual health or well-being and what role it plays in your life, but its significance is stronger than you may believe. Spiritual wellness may mean different things to different people. For some, spirituality may be synonymous with traditional religion, while for others it relates primarily to the quality of personal relationships or love for nature. A basic foundation for spiritual wellness may be the sense that life is meaningful and you have found your place in it. The search for meaning and purpose in human existence leads one to strive for a state of harmony with him/herself and with others while working to balance inner needs with the rest of the world.

Signs of Spiritual Wellness:

- Development of a purpose in life

- Ability to spend reflective time alone

- Taking time to reflect on the meaning of events in life

- Having a clear sense of right and wrong, and act accordingly

- Ability to explain why you believe what you believe

- Caring and acting for the welfare of others and the environment

- Being able to practice forgiveness and compassion in life

The human spirit is the most neglected aspect of our selves. Just as we exercise to condition our bodies, a healthy spirit is nurtured by purposeful practice. The spirit is the aspect of ourselves that can carry us through anything. If we take care of our spirit, we will be able to experience a sense of peace and purpose even when life deals us a severe blow. A strong spirit helps us to survive and thrive with grace, even in the face of difficulty.

Developing spiritual health generally begins with an individual's desire to give life purpose and meaning through the internal examination of their worldview. For example, some individuals believe in one higher power that intervenes in their life when they pray. Therefore, these individuals spend time praying every day or week in order to foster their spiritual health. Other individuals believe that meditation, or silent focus on their inner being, is necessary for finding a path to enlightenment that elevates their spiritual health for the duration of their lives.

Are you spiritually healthy? Ask yourself the following questions:

- Do you have a positive outlook on life?

- Do you feel a sense of serenity, peace or worth?

- Do you have a sense of purpose or meaning in your life?

- Do you have feelings of emptiness, anxiety, hopelessness or apathy?

- Do you face many conflicts in your life and keep ending up with the same negative thinking patterns or attracting the same kind of negative people into your life?

In case you feel more of the two last points it's time to reflect on your life, yourself and start improving your spiritual health. Identify a few things in your life that give you an inner peace, comfort, strength, love or connection. Things that can help you spiritually could be community service, volunteering, meditating, spending time in nature, yoga, tai chi, Reiki, singing, reading etc.

Start searching for the bigger picture. Start thinking outside of the box. Live joyfully, smile and laugh a lot. Be thankful and forgiving. Be open to new experiences, new people, new opportunities. It's the part of us that lets us find meaning in our life.

LIFE BALANCE

ensure you maintain a certain level of balance... spiritually, physically, emotionally, socially, mentally and financially. You need to balance work and family, and all the other areas of your life without spreading yourself too thin and having a guilt trip when you do one thing, but think you should be doing another.

All of the key areas of our lives overlap and interlink, effecting each other. Unless we create for ourselves satisfaction in each and every part of our life, we can never truly be fulfilled, or live a contented, happy and healthy life.

"No success in public life can compensate for failure in the home"

- Benjamin Disraeli (British Prime Minister)

CONCLUSION

By embracing a lifestyle filled with good health and fitness, the risk of contracting several diseases can be greatly reduced. Typical diseases that healthy individuals reduce the risk of contracting include diabetes, heart disease, several types of cancer, asthma and osteoporosis.

In addition, a healthy lifestyle also promotes lower blood pressure, reduces the likelihood of injuries and falls, and improves mental health and a sense of well-being. It is also beneficial in overcoming insomnia. In fact, even the length of one's life can be increased by adhering to a healthy and fit lifestyle.

Living a healthy lifestyle is beneficial in many ways. In fact, an individual who is healthy tends to feel more confident, and may feel more in control of their life.

In addition, the strength and stamina of that individual will increase, allowing them to participate in new activities. Living a lifestyle that is conducive to good health, fitness and mental well-being can reduce the probability of contracting numerous diseases and ailments and extend the length of one's life as well.

Turning Theory Into Practice

We've covered a lot of topics in this beginners guide, probably to the extent of overwhelming you with everything you need to be doing to achieve a healthy lifestyle. So how can you take all the pointers from this guide and incorporate them into your life quickly and effectively?

Well it's time to stop reading and instead, start doing! You may have already seen my Healthy Lifestyle Plan on Healthy Lifestyles Living. Now before I continue I just want to point out **this is not a sales pitch, I don't want any money from you, I want to make a difference and help you lead a healthy lifestyle. You can learn all the about the Healthy Lifestyle Plan and it won't cost you a penny!**

So what is The Healthy Lifestyle Plan? Well you've already read about it! It covers everything you need to know about all the concepts mentioned in this beginners guide. More importantly though, it's the way The Healthy Lifestyle Plan is delivered which makes it an easy to use yet highly effective healthy lifestyle program.

The process is simple. Every day I introduce a new healthy lifestyle concept, idea or topic. I will then give you all the information you need to know about the topic for the day and then give you a "habit challenge" which is a simple task that I ask you to perform for the day. Once the challenge has been set, you then need to incorporate the challenge into the next day and then the next day and so on. By receiving a new small challenge every single day, after the first 30 days, you will have made 30 small changes to your daily routine which will have had dramatic changes on your lifestyle, health and wellbeing.

Not only does it show you how to get healthy, it's incredibly fun to use and if you find yourself struggling at any time you can simply email me your questions or concerns and I will be on hand to give you my professional advice, tips and techniques to keep you going.

I include everything you need to keep your healthy lifestyle on track from a daily and weekly food scoring system to relaxation scripts and much more.

FULL DISCLAIMER: *The Healthy Lifestyle Plan is 100% free but if you wish to take advantage of our "done for you" support tools then we charge a small monthly fee. If you're prepared to download a few forms and keep your own health records or record your own relaxation scripts then you can do the plan for free. It's entirely up to you.*

To get started simply go to The Healthy Lifestyle Plan (https://www.healthylifestylesliving.com/healthy-lifestyle-plan/) and sign up now. You will need to enter your email address so I can send you the daily challenges. Rest assured that this is all I will send! I treat my subscribers' privacy and time with the upmost respect!

By providing your email address and opting in to my free Healthy Lifestyle Plan I will:

- Send you a daily email introducing the next healthy lifestyle concept, tip or advice.

- Answer any questions you send with regards to The Healthy Lifestyle Plan.

- Let you know about any changes to The Healthy Lifestyle Plan.

- Show you how to use the support tools and other resources available to you for The Healthy Lifestyle Plan (free and paid for options).

- Tell you about any other product, guide and/or blog post of my own that I think will be of great help to you on your healthy lifestyle journey.

- Include an unsubscribe link on every email I send you so you can opt-out of The Healthy Lifestyle Plan at any time if you wish to do so.

I will not

- Sell or share your email address with any third party. Period!

- Spam you with affiliate products or offers. Period!

So head on over to The Healthy Lifestyle Plan sign up page (https://www.healthylifestylesliving.com/healthy-lifestyle-plan/) now and I'll see you there!

Lastly, I do hope you have found this guide useful. If you know someone else who could also benefit from this guide then of course, send them a copy direct but I would really appreciate it if you could help me spread the word about this amazing free resource through any of our social media channels. Head on over to our Beginners Guide To A Healthy Lifestyle webpage (https://www.healthylifestylesliving.com/the-beginners-guide-to-a-healthy-lifestyle/) and hit the like and/or share button for your favourite social media sites to help us spread the Healthy Lifestyle message or feel free to leave a comment and let me know what you thought of this free guide.

If you're a website owner or just want to share the link to the book itself in an email or newsletter then please direct your audience to this link:

https://www.healthylifestylesliving.com/the-beginners-guide-to-a-healthy-lifestyle/

All that's left now is for me to wish you luck and if you're interested to tell you a bit more about my story. As a Health & Wellness Life Coach I want you to know that even my lifestyle hasn't always been healthy. No one is perfect - all we can do is make the best choice possible in the situations that are presented to us on this journey we call life.

Until next time,

Larry Lewis.

Health & Wellness Life Coach.
www.healthylifestylesliving.com

My (Brief) Story

I want to let you in on a little secret. At the time of reading this guide I am not healthy. Yes I have my reasons (or are they excuses) - problems with my eye led me to live a sedentary lifestyle etc etc but it was the choices I made at this time which were the reason for me to put on weight as I traded easiness and convenience over my health.

Why am I telling you this? I think it's important you know that even someone who has all the answers, knows exactly what needs to be done to live a healthy lifestyle, who has the same choices as you do can make the wrong decisions when it comes to their health given the right circumstances. It sounds so obvious but it's more important to live a healthy lifestyle than know how to live one. This is why I use my unique training method for my Healthy Lifestyle Plan. It makes sure you don't get bogged down in information and makes you take action.

2014 was a dark year for me, I went through bouts of depression yet there was one thing that kept me going - my passion to help others. It was Boxing Day morning in 2015 where I finally said 'No more, this isn't me, I can get through this.' Because the truth is I'm probably one of the most positive people you could ever meet. It is that that got me through every crisis I'd been through since my eye problems first started.

It was time to get back to living my life with a positive outlook and allow my knowledge of healthy lifestyle living to direct me. This was the beginning of a new path. I no longer was just writing about healthy lifestyles I was living it once again.

They say the road to recovery is a long one and although I'm not yet back at peak performance just yet, I'm well on my way to getting my healthy lifestyle back.

No matter where you are in life right now, take an example from my book for what **not to do**. Don't let life's problems de-rail you. Stay positive, learn and implement all the information in the Healthy Lifestyle Plan and start (or continue if you're one of the lucky ones) living life to the max.

This guide and the Healthy Lifestyle Plan is for everyone. Use it, have fun with it and enjoy all the benefits of being healthy. I am and within a very short time you can too.

www.ingramcontent.com/pod-product-compliance
Lightning Source LLC
Chambersburg PA
CBHW071249280526
45788CB00004B/1648